ORAL CARE FOR THE CANCER PATIENT

Kris Potts,
BS, FAADH, RDH

Table of Contents

This book is intended to provide general education and information related to oral care for patients undergoing cancer treatment. It is not a substitute for professional medical or dental advice, diagnosis, or treatment. Readers should consult qualified healthcare professionals for individual guidance.

Printed in the United States of America
First Edition

Cover Design: Isabella Brooks

(Fiverr: isabela_brooks)
Interior Formatting: Isabella Brooks

For more information or permissions, contact:

www.krispottsrdh.com krprdh79@gmail.com

PREFACE

Misty. She was one of the first people I loved who suffered from cancer that I can remember. She was my best friend for more than 35 years. Never in my wildest dreams, as we were doing life side by side, did I imagine I would lose her.

We met through our church youth group around 1970. However, we lived across town from each other and attended different schools, yet we never let that keep us from becoming the closest of friends. We both got married in 1977 and were honored to be part of each other's special day. In 1985, we each gave birth to daughters just five weeks apart. The girls, as different as night and day, grew up together and remained close to this day. So close, in fact, that they call each other sisters. In 1995, Misty's oldest sister, Pam, lost her battle with metastatic breast cancer. With her mother, father, and brother already gone, Misty was left with no immediate family—except for mine. We celebrated holidays together and supported each other through recitals, school awards, and life's many milestones.

Six years later, in 2001, Misty received devastating news: breast cancer. She was terrified after having witnessed her sister's journey. As a single parent with a limited income, she lacked the resources that Pam had—no health insurance, no emergency fund, no 401(k). She could not see a light at the end of the tunnel.

I promised to be by her side through it all, and I was. I had no idea what we were in for. First, there was the biopsy. That was the easy part. Surgery, reconstruction, and chemotherapy followed. I drove her to treatments, sat with her through procedures, and shaved her head when her hair began to fall out. We both cried that night.

She suffered agonizing mucositis, and as a dental hygienist, I felt helpless. I should have been able to do more to relieve her suffering. She had difficulty eating, swallowing, and speaking. She would cry from the pain. I had treated patients with aphthous ulcers over the years, but I had never seen anything like this. There were few products available for relief, and I knew only what the oncology team instructed.

Toward the end of 2004, the chemotherapy was over, the surgery had healed, and we thought we had the cancer beat. We were elated to be moving out of this nightmare. But Misty wasn't that lucky. On New Year's Eve, my phone rang. It was Misty's daughter, home for the holidays and looking forward to family celebrations, but what she told me would change our entire holiday season.

"Something is wrong with Mom, and I don't know what to do."

We decided it wasn't a 911 emergency, but she needed to get to the emergency room. My husband and I drove over to take them.

As you might imagine, the emergency room of the county hospital on New Year's Eve was a circus. At the time, I thought she had suffered a mild stroke, and that doctors would fix her up and everything would go back to normal.

After hours of waiting, the doctor finally spoke with us. My heart fell to the floor. I knew this was bad. The cancer was back, but this time in her lungs, liver, and brain, just like her sister's.

I became her planner, scheduler, power of attorney, patient advocate, and practical adult. Misty was an emotional wreck. The thing she feared the most was coming true: she would not be around experiencing the milestones in her daughter's life.

Misty introduced me to the world of cancer. Since then, I have served as a caregiver to varying degrees for my uncle (esophageal cancer), my brother-in-law (oral cancer), and my mother (pancreatic cancer). I am a breast cancer survivor myself. I've seen—and felt—the physical and emotional toll of oncology care. As a dental hygienist for over 30 years of my 40-plus years in dentistry, I've witnessed how cancer treatments affect the mouth: inflammation, dry mouth, rampant decay, and the heartbreaking resignation of "I survived cancer, now this."

I've seen the raw emotions, the anxiety, and the lack of compliance when patients don't understand the cancer journey. That's why I've dedicated myself to educating my colleagues. Consequently, I have been led to share this information with my colleagues so that, maybe, you, too, can help a loved one, patient, or family member who is going through a similar experience with their cancer diagnosis. I have spent countless hours researching products that claim to be the answer to dry mouth, how to prevent rampant decay, and studying the oral–systemic connection that often results in expensive oral rehabilitation. I developed continuing education courses and completed certification in oncology care. I have had the pleasure of lecturing internationally and authoring several journal and magazine articles on these topics.

I have come to understand that life is a journey. Situations that we don't expect happen all the time. We can let them define us, and we can also realize that these situations can create the path we take. Cancer has shaped my path, and for that, I am thankful because it is allowing me to make a difference in the world.

In the pages that follow, I share my Prehabilitation Concepts to help dental professionals have the tools they need to keep their patients' mouths healthy when the immune system is compromised by cancer treatment. These concepts can be implemented right away, whether readers are dental professionals, caregivers, family members of a cancer patient, or patients themselves. I hope that Dental Practitioners become better equipped to understand the journey and become a resource for cancer patients. Our profession can do more than pat their arm and express our condolences. We must move beyond making blanket recommendations for outdated products that only provide palliative relief and detrimentally affect the dentition.

CHAPTER 1

DIAGNOSIS: UNDERSTANDING THE CANCER JOURNEY

Cancer doesn't discriminate. It doesn't matter about age, gender, race, or social status. It affects not only the diagnosed person but also their family, friends, and caregivers. As dental professionals, we often see patients more frequently than their primary care providers. That gives us a unique opportunity to support them not just clinically, but emotionally.

This chapter explores what patients, and their loved ones are going through. It's about empathy, awareness, and being prepared to meet them where they are at.

This book does not focus solely on the effects of oral cancer. Cancer that occurs *anywhere* in the body affects the oral cavity. With any cancer diagnosis, patients are advised to obtain dental clearance before beginning treatment, and this is the ideal time to engage in the process of prehabilitation. Research notes prehabilitative oral care provided by a dentist is associated with a decreased incidence of postoperative pneumonia and death within 30 days following oncology surgery (Ishimaru et al., 2018). Oral infections can complicate cancer treatment outcomes.

Dental professionals can help patients recognize discrepancies between public opinion and evidence-based recommendations. Patients newly diagnosed with cancer are often inundated with recommendations about alternative medicines and cures. These suggestions usually come from well-meaning friends, family members, and even random acquaintances—sometimes before the patient has even asked for advice. Turning to "Dr. Google" for answers often leads to misinformation. While people shouldn't expect a website to replace a medical professional, they usually do. This leaves health care providers with the task of helping patients sort through and identify misinformation and provide education without judgment. Development of a network of colleagues for referrals, i.e., dieticians/nutritional therapists, mental health counselors, Myofunctional Therapists, sharing information regarding local support groups, and encouraging them to ask their oncologist about clinical trials are all ways to support our patients.

Educational brochures on products, human papillomavirus, cancer risk factors, and the rise in oral cancer are additional ways to get vital, factual information into patients' hands, but be cautious about simply handing out a stack of brochures: they will likely end up in the trash. Instead, ask the patient if they would like more information about a specific topic and then provide it. If a dental professional feels confident in their ability to provide direct support and guidance, they could offer that and provide their office number for the patient to contact them.

The Emotional Journey

When someone hears the words "you have cancer", their world changes instantly. Their emotional response often follows the following five stages:

1. Denial – Shock, disbelief, and numbness.
2. Anger – Frustration, blame, and resentment occur when the patient or family members can no longer deny the reality of the situation.
3. Bargaining – With doctors, with God, with fate.
4. Depression – Grief, fear, and emotional exhaustion.
5. Acceptance – A new sense of reality and purpose.

Patients often enter "survival mode," pushing aside their emotions to focus on treatment. Still, feelings don't disappear, they resurface later, sometimes in unexpected sentiments such as "I can't worry about that right now" or "I'm in a fight for my life."
Patients often try to restore balance amid the chaos that has suddenly become their existence. During active treatment, they become so busy with appointments and procedures that it can take a while for their mind and body to catch up. Many begin to embrace mindfulness by living more in the moment and adjusting their perspective. They re-evaluate priorities and don't sweat the small stuff, realizing it's all small stuff. Over time, they also tend to reject negativity in their surroundings.

There is a grieving process for what will never be—the loss of abilities, the loss of body parts, the loss of life—and even a fear of death. All these feelings can lead to clinical depression or an inability to experience either pain or pleasure, leaving patients feeling emotionally numb. Scars and adhesions can contribute to a distorted body image, and there is often an underlying fear of recurrence, coupled with anxiety about passing the disease on to future generations.

When I go for my mammogram, there's always a moment of scanxiety—a form of post-traumatic stress. I don't realize I am holding my breath and tensing my body until I'm told that nothing's changed, everything looks fine, I'm good to go, until next year. Only then can I breathe again.

That fear never completely goes away. Every lump, every twinge, every pain carries the possibility of recurrence (Gubar, 2018). There is also the fear of genetic legacy. Many survivors worry about passing cancer on to their children. Genetic testing can offer reassurance, but fear often lingers.

I was very fortunate that my cancer was small, noninvasive, caught early, and that the best of all possible outcomes occurred at every step throughout treatment. But others are not so lucky. I had genetic testing done because I wanted to know whether there was anything my daughter needed to be aware of as she got older. The results were favorable, but even so, the emotional weight and underlying fear remain.

Posts on social media show people "ringing the bell" at the end of radiation treatment or holding up a sign that reads "last chemo appointment." However, the journey is not over just because the treatment is.

CHAPTER 2

THE HIDDEN EMOTIONAL TOLL

Post-traumatic stress disorder (PTSD) in a cancer patient presents differently than in other trauma populations, nor may it always manifest as full-blown PTSD. In a cancer patient, PTSD tends to be more momentary and affects the caregivers and family members who are also at risk. Approximately 40% of patients with cancer experience significant emotional and social distress during treatment (Pranjic et al., 2016), with approximately one-third of patients developing distress that requires specialized intervention (Grassi et al., 2017).

An example I personally experienced occurred during my first appointment with my oncologist. I had not been to their office before, and I punched in the address in my GPS. I froze in the parking lot. It was the same building where Misty had her treatments. I was not sure I could walk in. However, as it turned out, a new building had been built right behind the old one, and it now housed the oncology center. I was relieved. Certain smells, sounds, or anniversaries can be emotional triggers resulting in panic attacks, emotional outbursts, and survivors' guilt. Other symptoms of PTSD can manifest in excessive fitness routines and hyperfocus on nutrition and ingredients of products. Be prepared to answer questions about ingredients in everyday products we use, as the patient may want to avoid certain ones.

Cancer affects more than the patient—it reshapes the lives of caregivers too. Whether they are administering medications, managing appointments, or simply offering emotional support, caregivers often experience burnout, isolation, vicarious trauma, along with guilt and helplessness. Many times, they suppress their own grief and exhaustion.

Cancer can be isolating for patients, even if they have many people around to support them. Some might feel lonely because their family and friends have trouble understanding and coping with their diagnosis, and some may lack a family safety net. As previously mentioned, when Misty's older sister Pam lost her battle with metastatic breast cancer, Misty had no family left except her daughter, myself, my husband and our daughter.

Caregivers today are asked to participate in more procedures than ever before, including administering oral treatments and home-based chemotherapies, caring for patients' access ports and lines for medication delivery and blood draws, managing pain medications, and monitoring patient well-being. These medical complexities, along with the emotional worry and distress that come with a cancer diagnosis and the potential physical and cognitive declines of the patient, make cancer caregiving extremely stressful.

Some family members and friends serve as direct caregivers, while others take on supporting roles by helping with meals or childcare after school, and still others provide support from a distance.

The stress and feeling of isolation often lead caregivers to turn to unhealthy coping mechanisms, while others use different strategies (Familycaregiveronline, 2023). Regardless of their role, each person's contribution has a meaningful impact on the patients and their loved ones' well-being. This is their "new normal." Nearly 90% of people who survive a traumatic event experience guilt (Amenclinics.com, 2021). As a provider, your role is not to fix it—but to acknowledge it, validate it, and walk alongside them as a caregiver.

Even just saying, "You are doing a great job," can mean the world.

- Cancer is not just a physical disease; it is an emotional and psychological journey.
- Dental professionals are uniquely positioned to support patients and caregivers.
- Empathy, education, and presence can make a profound difference in the emotional health of a patient or caregiver.
- Understanding the emotional landscape of cancer helps us provide better, more compassionate care.

CHAPTER 3

A CANCER OVERVIEW

To provide adequate care for patients undergoing cancer treatment, dental professionals must understand the disease itself. This chapter offers a concise overview of different types of cancer, how cancer is classified, and the treatments patients may undergo—each of which has significant oral implications.

When cancer is suspected, there are three possible biopsy outcomes:

1. **Benign.** This is the most common outcome and indicates that the lesion is noncancerous and not life-threatening.

2. **Premalignant (epithelial dysplasia).** In this case, the cells forming the epithelial layers appear abnormal (atypical). Dysplasia is graded as mild, moderate, or severe, depending on the number of dysplastic cells observed. When dysplastic lesions such as lichen planus are found in the mouth, removal is not always necessary. Regardless

of treatment decisions, close and regular follow-up is essential to monitor any visual changes at the lesion site. Premalignant lesions can recur, and malignant transformation remains possible at any time.

3. **Carcinoma in situ.** This diagnosis indicates that atypical cells are present throughout the epithelial layers but have not penetrated the basement membrane into the connective tissue. Once cells breach the basement membrane, the lesion is classified as invasive cancer (Czerninski et al., 2008).

Cancer is often described by its stage and grade, for example, stage IV, high grade. Staging and grading provide a common language for communicating clinical information among medical professionals. This shared terminology aids in treatment planning, prognosis, outcome evaluation, and the exchange of information between treatment centers.

Grading refers to how closely cancer cells resemble a normal cell from the same anatomical site when viewed under a microscope.

- Low grade: Cells appear more normal, slower growing.
- High grade: Cells appear very abnormal, more aggressive.

Staging is determined by the TNM system (tumor/node/metastasis), which has been the standard classification system for solid cancers since the 1980s:

- T – Size and location of primary tumor
- N – Degree of lymph node involvement
- M – Presence of metastasis

Note: Blood cancers and pediatric cancers use different staging systems.

Stage categories:

- 0 – Carcinoma in situ
- I, II, III – Increasing tumor size and lymph node involvement

- IV – Metastasis to other organs

Cancer Treatment Modalities and Oral Implications

There are **seven main treatment options** for cancer. Each has unique oral side effects that dental professionals must be prepared to manage.

1. **Chemotherapy**. Chemotherapy uses combinations of toxic drugs to kill or shrink cancer cells. Unfortunately, these agents also damage healthy cells. Many of these drug cocktails are so potent that nurses must be careful when handling them. The side effects are often severe: in addition to hair loss, many patients lose their fingernails, eyelashes, and eyebrows. They develop blisters on their feet and hands, as well as ulcer-like sores on their faces and in their mouths. Oral complications such as mucositis, burning tongue, and widespread dentition breakdown are common. It is a heart-wrenching experience for patients to endure chemotherapy and then face the aftereffects.

"I sat with Misty during her infusions. Some patients had friends. Some were alone. Some cried the whole time. It was heartbreaking. Moreover, the oral side effects—blisters, ulcers, burning tongue—were devastating."

2. **Hormone therapy.** Hormone therapies either block the body's ability to produce hormones or interfere with how those hormones behave in the body. They are commonly used to treat cancers that depend on hormones for growth and are often administered concurrently with other cancer treatments.

3. **Surgical treatment.** Surgery can be disfiguring or functionally limiting, affecting speech, swallowing, and the ability to maintain oral hygiene. While some surgical scars are hidden from view, they remain visible to the patient long after treatment is complete.

4. **Bone marrow/stem cell transplants.** These procedures are generally used to treat

blood cancers such as leukemia. Because patients undergo intensive chemotherapy and radiation prior to the transplant to improve the likelihood of success, 70–90% develop oral mucositis or stomatitis as a result (Nagagaki et al., 2022).

5. **Targeted therapy.** These therapies use drugs that target specific genes, proteins, or receptors involved in the growth and survival of cancer cells. These genes regulate how cells produce the proteins essential to keep cells working. If genes mutate, the proteins change too, which can cause cells to divide excessively and allow them to live much longer than they should. When this happens, the cells grow out of control and form a tumor. Although targeted therapy produces fewer side effects than chemo, it can still affect oral tissues.

6. **Radiation therapy.** For head and neck cancers, a custom-fitted mask is made, and the targeted areas are carefully marked. During each treatment, the patient is secured to the

table with a mask to ensure the area remains immobile and that radiation consistently reaches the intended site. For other parts of the body, semi-permanent "tattoos" may be used for alignment and accuracy. Radiation has residual effects regardless of where it is targeted on the body. It can cause xerostomia, mucositis, and osteoradionecrosis. Brachytherapy, a type of radiotherapy, involves placing tiny radioactive "seeds" within the targeted area. Patients treated with brachytherapy have a higher risk of developing osteonecrosis of the jaw.

7. **Immunotherapy.** Immunotherapeutics are a class of drugs currently approved to treat several types of cancers, including melanoma and lung cancer. It is often used in cases of rapidly progressing head and neck cancers. It has been shown to double survival rates while producing fewer side effects, thereby improving patients' quality of life. Immunotherapeutics have also been shown to be highly effective in patients with tumors that are human papillomavirus (HPV)- positive. The number of

head and neck cancers attributable to HPV infection has increased by approximately 250% over the past several decades (Mayo, L., 2017). Although immunotherapy has about one-third the rate of serious side effects, it can still result in the following:

- Injection site pain
- Rash
- Fatigue
- Nausea, diarrhea, constipation
- Flu-like symptoms

Immunotherapy has also doubled the number of patients whose tumors have shrunk and increased the number of patients who, after six months of treatment, have shown no progression of the disease.

Universal Oral Impacts of Cancer Treatments

Regardless of what type of therapy is used, *all* treatments can:

- Suppress the immune system

- Affect blood glucose levels
- Feed oral bacteria
- Build biofilm
- Cause xerostomia
- Alter oral pH

When we put these together, they contribute to increased rates of decay, more complicated dental procedures, and delayed healing.

- ❖ Understanding cancer staging and treatment helps dental professionals anticipate oral complications.
- ❖ Each treatment modality has unique oral side effects that require tailored care.
- ❖ Dental providers play a critical role in identifying, managing, and preventing complications.

CHAPTER 4

ORAL COMPLICATIONS OF CANCER TREATMENT

Cancer treatments do not just affect the body, they profoundly impact on the mouth (Raber-Durlache et al., 2004). As dental professionals, we are often the first to recognize and manage these complications. Understanding the oral side effects of cancer therapies enables us to prevent pain, preserve dental function, and improve our patients' quality of life.

The most widespread complication in oncology patients is xerostomia and hyposalivation. Severe xerostomia is seen more frequently in patients who have head and neck cancer and have been treated with radiation therapy. Xerostomia is defined as the subjective feeling of a dry mouth. Hyposalivation is the objective measure of a decreased salivary flow rate. The term "dry mouth" is often used to describe both (Islas-Granillo et al., 2017).

Xerostomia can occur with doses of radiation as low as 10 grays, with permanent hyposalivation occurring at doses greater than 25 gray. Intensity-modulated radiation therapy (IMRT) has dramatically reduced collateral damage to the salivary glands. However, patients who underwent conventional cone-beam or fixed-field radiation typically experience more severe xerostomia.

The serous glands are often more impaired than the mucous glands, resulting in viscous, ropy saliva with an acidic pH and, in turn, impaired tooth remineralization. Have you heard of extracting salivary glands and reimplanting them after treatment? It is a controversial approach, but you could be asked about it. The primary concern is that the proximity of the glands to the original tumor site may increase the risk of malignant cell dissemination. Because of the rapid cell turnover of most oral cancers, one of those pesky cancer cells could likely enter the bloodstream or lymphatic system during the procedure.

Patients experiencing moderate to severe xerostomia after treatment often develop an intolerance to oral medications, necessitating the use of other delivery forms such as liquids or transdermal patches. These patients are at increased risk for mucosal injury, fungal infections (most commonly candidiasis), and rampant dental decay due to the lack of salivary protective factors. They may also be unable to wear their removable partials and dentures comfortably.

To support oral health, consider evaluating salivary pH and composition. Are you currently using salivary diagnostic testing chairside? This testing is rapidly evolving as a tool for both screening and diagnostics and has become an important adjunct for dental professionals (UCSF School of Dentistry, n.d.). These tests can provide valuable information on caries risk, salivary flow rates, salivary pH, and periodontal pathogens. They can also quantify bacterial load and identify which microorganisms are active in the biofilm. Promising research suggests that salivary proteins from certain cancers can be detected in saliva, enabling earlier detection.

Another condition frequently encountered in patients undergoing oncology treatment is osteonecrosis, which is typically seen in patients treated with bisphosphonate therapy (Estillo et al., 2008). ALL health care professionals should be aware of a patient's history of bisphosphonate use, as these medications have a half-life of 15 years or longer! Some bisphosphonates can cause long-term effects, even if they were used only once in the past. Even a short-term uptake of one to two months can cause complications. It is important to ask whether the patient has ever been treated with these medications. There are some newer drugs (Aredia™, Xgeva™, Prolia™) that allow for a "drug holiday "for emergent dental treatments, such as extractions. Temporarily discontinuing their use provides a 1- to 2-week window for dental treatment. This, of course, requires consultation and coordination with the oncology team.

Medication-Related Osteonecrosis of the Jaw

Medically related osteonecrosis (MRONJ) has been added to the lexicon because of tyrosine kinase inhibitors (TKIs) found in drugs other than bisphosphonates (Sutent™, Avastin™). TKIs block the cellular signals that promote growth and division during the cell cycle. TKIs also block the growth of new blood vessels (angiogenesis), thereby starving cancer cells and activating oncogenes. TKIs are an example of targeted therapy and can result in osteonecrosis. In addition, commonly used immunosuppressive and antiarthritis drugs were used to treat patients with COVID-19 during the height of the pandemic. While these drugs showed a significantly lower mortality rate in patients with COVID-19, these drugs may also put the patients treated for COVID with these drugs at higher risk of developing medication-related osteonecrosis of the jaw (Hasan, 2021)

MRONJ is seen more often in males, more often in the mandible, and can occur spontaneously, not just after a trauma. On presentation, the patient often complains of jaw pain or numbness, or a feeling that the jaw is "heavy." On assessment, the practitioner needs to look for loosening of any teeth or exposed areas of bone in the mouth and conduct an external examination as well. If the patient presents with swelling, redness, or drainage outside the oral cavity, *look inside the oral cavity*. This can be an external presentation of osteonecrosis. Often, medical professionals do not look *inside* the patient's mouth to determine the possible source!

Mucositis is the painful inflammation and ulceration of the mucous membranes, commonly triggered by chemotherapy or radiation. It is one of the most debilitating side effects of cancer treatment and significantly impacts a patient's quality of life. Mucositis compels aggressive treatment for pain management. The dental professional needs to keep in mind that these lesions are not the garden-variety aphthous ulcers! These ulcers serve as portals for opportunistic bacterial, viral, and fungal infections, including herpes simplex, herpes zoster (shingles), candida, and cytomegalovirus.

The onset of mucositis occurs between 2 and 14 days after the first chemo infusion. It is sometimes referred to as CTOM (chemotherapy-induced oral mucositis) and can occur anywhere along the gastrointestinal tract, not just in the oral cavity. If severe enough, it can necessitate a stoppage of chemotherapy and an increased use of pain medications, increased tube feedings, and longer stays in the hospital (Laheij et al., 2014).

Treatment Challenges and Misconceptions

Dentistry's "Windex," CHX (chlorahexidine), is ineffective against mucositis. There is also a product commonly recommended called "Magic Mouthwash." There is no uniform formula for the compounding of Magic Mouthwash, and the suspension that is prepared usually contains high levels of sucrose, which, of course, contributes to decay. Yes, it will numb the pain, but studies show there is no difference in the severity, onset, or duration of ulcers compared with sterile saline rinses.

"Misty called it pond scum. She suffered more than she should have because she could not tolerate it."

Cryotherapy may be used to prevent mucositis by having the patient suck on ice chips or hold ice water in their mouth before, during, and/or after infusions of systemic therapies commonly associated with mucositis. The application of cold causes vasoconstriction, which limits the amount of the drug that reaches the oral tissues and reduces the risk of mouth sores (Mayo Clinic Staff, 2004). Studies have shown that this approach is highly effective for patients. You may also have seen patients use cold caps; a form of cryotherapy that helps prevent hair loss during chemotherapy. When cryotherapy is applied intraorally, patients experience significantly fewer oral symptoms, less difficulty eating and drinking, shorter symptom duration, and a less significant impact on their quality of life (Swarm et al., 2019).

Alternative Therapies and Cannabinoids

Nearly 40% of patients feel that cancer can be cured through "alternative" therapies, such as oxygen therapy, diet, and herbs, without standard cancer treatments. Certain drug cocktails are more likely to cause nausea and vomiting than others. Many turn to the use of medicinal marijuana to alleviate the nausea and vomiting that come with most treatments (Zhang, 2018). Marijuana contains two major phytocannabinoids: cannabidiol (CBD) and tetrahydrocannabinol (THC). CBD activates receptors in the brain that reduce fear and psychological stress responses, whereas THC regulates fear and anxiety-related behaviors (Harrison & Barclay, 2018).

Did you know we have a vomiting center in our brain? The THC in marijuana is believed to relieve nausea via the reflex pathways acting as receptors, reversing the effects of serotonin receptors in the brain. Proposed medicinal uses of cannabis include analgesic and antiemetic effects in patients with cancer, reduction of anxiety and depression in patients with post-traumatic stress disorder (PTSD), and adjunctive therapy for neuropathic pain in patients with chronic pain syndromes. When using familiar standard scoring systems to evaluate pain and discomfort, the use of marijuana has been shown to decrease anxiety, depression, pain, and discomfort while increasing the feelings of general well-being and improved quality of life. Many believe that the use of cannabinoids will become part of the standard of care in treating cancer patients' anxiety and pain (Harrison & Barclay, 2018).

Long-Term Post Treatment Effects

The long-term post treatment effects of cancer treatment can include sleep disorders, eating disorders, and altered smell and taste that affect nutritional consumption. Specific therapies may increase cravings for high-sugar foods and carbohydrates. Other long-term post treatment effects in patients include reduced libido, residual joint pain, and difficulty concentrating when reading books or documents. They have difficulty with cognitive and emotional changes, including verbalization and communication. Many patients experience short-term memory loss, commonly referred to as "chemo brain," which can affect simple daily tasks, such as remembering how to turn on the television or use a light switch. These effects can lead to difficulty making treatment decisions, evaluating alternative treatments, and maintaining compliance and participation in oral care. Post treatment complications can include accelerated bone density loss and neuropathy, which occurs in approximately 40% of treated patients (mskcc.org, 2022). Neuropathy can result in balance deficits and increase the risk of falls. In addition, some patients experience permanent heart and lung damage following radiotherapy for breast cancer, particularly if the cancer was located on the left side near the chest wall.

- Oral complications from cancer treatment are common, painful, and often preventable.
- Dental professionals must be proactive in identifying and managing these issues.
- Empathy, education, and collaboration with oncology teams are essential.

- Your role can dramatically improve a patient's comfort, confidence, and quality of life.

CHAPTER 5

PREHABILITATION CONCEPTS: PROACTIVE ORAL CARE BEFORE CANCER TREATMENT

Prehabilitation refers to comprehensive, proactive oral care provided *before* cancer treatment begins to address potential issues and minimize side effects as they develop. For cancer patients, this means preparing the oral environment before treatment begins—when the immune system is still intact, and healing is more predictable. As dental professionals, we can reduce complications, prevent pain, and even improve patient survival rates by acting early.

Prehabilitation concepts ideally occur in the window between diagnosis and the beginning of treatment, but they can be implemented at any time. It is an opportunity to decrease treatment-related morbidities and improve outcomes (Silver & Baima, 2013), establish baseline functional levels, provide targeted interventions, and decrease visits to the emergency department.

Best practices to reduce emergency department visits include identifying patients at high risk for unplanned acute care, enhancing access to and coordination of care across multiple providers, standardizing clinical pathways for symptom management, and early palliative care (Handley et al., 2018). By implementing early palliative care, the hospital readmission rate was reduced by nearly 50%, lowering overall healthcare costs for patients and the healthcare system. Moreover, prehabilitation concepts enable dental professionals to play a vital role in improving outcomes for patients diagnosed with cancer by increasing survival potential, educating patients and caregivers, and coordinating care with the oncology team.

A Japanese study of patients who underwent surgical treatment for head and neck, esophageal, gastric, colorectal, lung, or liver cancer between May 2012 and December 2015 found that preoperative oral care had a profound effect on postoperative complications after major cancer surgery (Ishimaru et al., 2018). Advances in diagnostics and both curative and palliative treatments have increased the number of individuals surviving cancer, and many are now using local resources for more of their health care needs. Consequently, the demand for dental professionals trained to meet the oral health care needs of both patients' battling cancer and cancer survivors is rising.

Barriers to Prehabilitation

Prehabilitation concepts come with obstacles, one of the biggest being the medical-dental disconnect.

"During my oncology certification, I heard nurses say, 'We do not tell patients everything—they will not do the treatment.'"

That is not informed consent. That is fear-based care. We can do better!

Within the medical community, there can sometimes be an attitude of "What do dentists know?" "They are not 'real' doctors" because they are outside of the "medical silo." Many dental professionals feel excluded or undervalued by the medical community. In addition, medical specialists often assume patients cannot afford dental treatment alongside oncology treatments. While many oncologists are brilliant in their field, they may not fully recognize the impact of oral health on treatment outcomes or how oral conditions can affect patients' daily functioning and overall quality of life. Some assume dental care is cosmetic or optional, while others fear overwhelming patients with too much information. This reflects a broader need for greater integration between medical and dental disciplines to support truly comprehensive patient care.

Systemic and Cultural Barriers

Many cancer treatment facilities lack on-site dental professionals, mainly because the medical community has historically failed to recognize the oral–systemic connection. That climate is beginning to change, thank goodness. There are obstacles to reimbursement, a lack of available information on intercollaboration, a shortage of role models in the field, and resistance to changing the status quo within the broader culture of health care, which has traditionally emphasized autonomy over collaboration. Professions need to shift their focus toward collaboration, partnerships, and sharing information. With a projected shortage of health care providers, including doctors and nurses, it will become imperative for interprofessional practices to work more collaboratively and efficiently (Vega & Bernard, 2017; Gregoriou et al., 2025).

Patient-Centered Barriers

There are also patient obstacles to implementing prehabilitation concepts. Many patients' undergoing cancer treatment are unaware that outcomes can be complicated by oral infections (e.g., periodontal disease, abscessed teeth, etc.). Because they are often in survival mode, the mouth is frequently the least of their concerns. Patients may also feel intimidated by their oncologist or overwhelmed by their circumstances, leading to hesitation or a fear of asking questions.

Limited patient access and insurance coverage often results from many individuals lacking an established dental home. Even when a dental referral *is* made, they experience challenges in obtaining timely appointments for a dental exam. It is not appropriate to tell a newly diagnosed cancer patient in need of prehabilitative care that your next available appointment is six to eight weeks away. These patients should be treated as urgent cases and scheduled for an appointment as soon as possible.

Financial concerns also exist. Approximately 57% of patients say that if faced with a cancer diagnosis, they would be concerned about the financial impact it would have on their families and about paying for treatment. Over 60% reported that they had resorted to drastic measures to help meet the cost of treatment, including early withdrawal from a retirement account, savings account, or college fund, taking out a second mortgage or other loan, postponing retirement, working additional hours, getting a second job, or even selling family heirlooms and other assets (Banbridge et al., 2011).

- Prehabilitation is proactive, preventive, and powerful.
- Dental professionals play a critical role in preparing patients for cancer treatment.
- Intercollaboration is essential to bridge the gap between medicine and dentistry.
- With education, empathy, and urgency, we can change the trajectory of a patient's journey.

CHAPTER 6

INTERCOLLABORATION: BRIDGING THE MEDICAL-DENTAL DIVIDE

Intercollaboration is defined as "multiple health workers from different professional backgrounds working together with patients, families, caregivers, and communities to deliver the highest quality of care." Intercollaborative efforts are critical to improving outcomes in cancer care (Gregoriou et al., 2025).

"In 2005, when I began this research, intercollaboration was unheard of. If we had had it during Misty's journey, it would have made everything easier."

We should actively develop professional relationships with oncologists, ear, nose, and throat specialists, oral surgeons, and other medical professionals. It involves:

- Mutual respect and shared goals
- Open communication
- Coordinated treatment planning
- A patient-centered approach

"Who doesn't love a basket of goodies? It's not about marketing—it's about connection."

Establishing the connection between dental and medical providers can be simple, elaborate, or somewhere in between. It can be as straightforward as dropping by with a business card or care kit and letting the oncology team know that your office is available for consultation and focused on the needs of their patients. Despite the clear connection between oral and systemic health, dentistry is often left out of the cancer care conversation, and patients suffer as a result, experiencing preventable complications, delayed healing, and a reduced quality of life. Intercollaboration is the solution.

"It's not about who's in charge—it's about what's best for the patient."

Once collaborative relationships are established, prehabilitation concepts can be so practical! Medical and dental providers can offer more personalized care by contributing to the development of reliable, internet-based resources and by creating systems that directly connect health care providers with survivors who are experiencing complications related to their diagnosis and treatment.

What do an electrical contractor, a chemist working in a laboratory, and a football player have in common? They all work in a team. Whether it is building a house, running a critical experiment, or winning a championship, these individuals rely on their team to reinforce their work and move it toward a greater goal. Interprofessional collaboration occurs when health care providers learn about each other's roles and responsibilities to coordinate care more effectively, reduce the likelihood of errors, and create a patient-centered rather than doctor-centered system. It can address complex ethical challenges and lead to improved outcomes, better care experience, and reduced health care costs.

There has long been a disconnect between oral health care and general health care. A multidisciplinary team of providers is needed to proactively address and treat pain and the side effects of cancer treatment adequately. It requires a team that includes a mouth care specialist (Nelson & Vega, 2018). Approximately

65% of medical offices report having no information, such as pamphlets or website links, to facilitate referrals to dentists (Atchison, 2018).

Approximately 90% of medical practices prefer electronic referrals over paper systems. Dental has not yet developed an electronic health care referral program due to the cost, especially for solo practitioners. It has been suggested that an app be developed at the federal/state/province level by a professional organization such as the ADA, allowing doctors to contact dentists, triage patients, and schedule appointments (Falvo, 2017). Lack of access to patient medical records limits coordination. Over half of doctors reported not referring a patient to a dentist in the past year because of inadequate dental referral systems. In the meantime, we can work on building those relationships.

The Importance of Follow-Up

So, you see an abnormality in the mouth. What do you do? You follow up! A lack of follow-up can carry significant liability implications.

"Misty lived paycheck to paycheck, with no insurance.

I don't recall any calls from her providers encouraging her to follow up. I wonder if her journey might have been different."

It is essential and very easy to do; it is as simple as sending an email or text or making a phone call. The following is an example dialogue that illustrates how this interaction might occur over the phone:

Office: "Ms. Smith, when you were in the other day, Dr. B found an abnormality that he was really concerned about. Did you see the oral surgeon we referred you to over on South Street? We were just curious if you had gone in."

Patient: "Oh, no. I have not been over there yet. I have not had time. He is not in my network."

Office: "Can we help you find a surgeon that is in your network? Can we maybe refer you to somebody closer to your work, so you do not have to drive across town to go see them?"

After the call, document a follow-up contact was made with the patient.

The optimal strategy would be to catch them before they walk out the door the same day they were in for their exam, but this is not always possible. I am unaware of any nursing or dental software systems currently in use that do not have the feature to flag follow-up with patients, either in their charts, on the schedule, or in the clinical notes. With most patient engagement systems, a message can be sent to notify patients that they missed a re-evaluation appointment.

However, many patients disregard these messages or reminders because they are busy, forget them, or consider them not serious. Few dental offices have established protocols for communicating with oncology teams, and many providers remain unfamiliar with interprofessional care models.

Be proactive. Do not wait for referrals. Reach out.

Legal and Ethical Considerations

In any case where a patient seeks legal counsel for a lack of referral or a missed diagnosis, an attorney will first examine whether documentation exists for both the screening and any follow-up. Simply stating you did it and that these steps were completed is not sufficient. The failure to refer—particularly when a clinician relies on their "biopsy eyes" (Cotton, 2021) and determines there is no need for the patient to see a surgeon or be evaluated further—is enormous. That is what an attorney is going to look for, anything that's going to result in a delayed diagnosis for that patient.

- Dental professionals must take the lead in building bridges.
- Intercollaboration is essential for comprehensive cancer care.
- Communication, education, and persistence are key.
- When we work together, patients win.

CHAPTER 7

ORAL ABNORMALITY SCREENING: A PROTOCOL FOR PREVENTION

Cancer patients face unique oral health challenges. Without a clear, proactive protocol, dental professionals may miss critical opportunities to prevent complications. In dentistry, thoughts automatically turn to oral cancers. Approximately 75% of all head and neck cancers begin in the oral cavities, and research shows that approximately 75% of all oral and oropharyngeal cancers are related to alcohol and tobacco use, including vaping (oralcancerfoundation.org, 2025). Oral and oropharyngeal cancers are both commonly referred to as oral cancer.

Cancer-causing infections such as human papillomavirus (HPV) and hepatitis are responsible for nearly 30% of cancer cases, amounting to over 450,000 new cases diagnosed each year (oralcancerfoundation.org, 2025). Every hour, every day, every week, of every month, of every year, one person dies from oral cancer. Only 57% of oral cancer patients, on average, will survive five years (oralcancerfoundation.org, 2025). That is the worst statistic of all cancer and has not changed in decades! This is mainly because most oral cancers are discovered at a late stage. For individuals who survive an initial oral cancer diagnosis, the risk of developing a second primary cancer is 20 times higher, most often occurring within the head and neck area, lungs, and esophagus. Younger, nonsmoking patients under the age of 50 are the fastest-growing oral cancer population. This is due to HPV replacing tobacco as the primary causative agent.

Does your office have a protocol when it comes to performing an oral abnormality screening? Is it a written protocol, or are you just expected to know? Is it followed? Does the Tuesday and Thursday hygienist follow the same criteria as the full-time hygienist? You may have a co-hygienist who does not place the same value on this screening as you do. If you do not have a written office protocol, this is an opportunity for you to develop one. By putting your current protocol in writing, you can share it with new hires, assistants, and even front office personnel. Front office staff can be our biggest allies—or our biggest obstacles—in implementing protocols.

What do you call this exam? A cancer screening? A cancer exam? Oral abnormality screening? I prefer oral abnormality screening because the abnormalities detected or assessed are lumps, bumps, or unusual appearances. Begin the screening by observing as you are bringing the patient back to the clinic area. Look for any asymmetry or swelling in the neck, discolored, ulcerated, or pigmented areas of skin, including the hair-bearing regions of the face and scalp. Despite objections of having 'hat hair', everyone should remove hats and caps when in the dental chair for this reason.

Listen to the patient's voice. Hoarseness lasting more than 2 weeks could indicate a more serious condition. A patient's symptoms and history will often lead the practitioner not only to the presence of a possible cancer, but also to the likely site of a lesion.

Utilize Motivational Interviewing

Ask the patient questions such as: “Have you noticed any changes in swallowing?” “Do things seem to stick or catch in your throat when you swallow?” “Have you noticed or felt any small lumps on the side of your neck while putting on makeup or shaving?” Most people tend to ignore subtle symptoms such as these, especially since they are not painful. However, these symptoms may indicate metastasis of oropharyngeal cancer from the primary site inside the mouth to the lymph nodes of the neck.

Ask patients to stick out their tongue and say “ahhh,” followed by questions such as: “Have you noticed changes in how your tongue moves?” “Can you stick your tongue out straight, without it veering to the side?” “Have you noticed any changes in your speech?” Oral cancers can affect the nerves that control tongue movement and speech articulation. Although often painless, these changes may subtly alter speech.

Overcoming Barriers to Oral Abnormality Screening: Fear and Language Matter

Many dental offices avoid using the word “cancer” out of concern for alarming patients. Reframing the examination as an oral abnormality screening might be less “scary” to the patient. Many offices do not perform such screenings. How important is it to you and your practice to provide this service? Oral abnormality screening is, in fact, a required component of a comprehensive dental examination.

Time Constraints and Practice Pressures

In an online research survey I conducted in 2018, the main reason cited for not performing an oral abnormality screening was a lack of time. We know our days are crammed. There is so much we are expected to do as dental professionals, even as appointment times are continually being shortened.

When evaluating success, consider other factors beyond production numbers, such as marketability. There are significant intangible benefits of being able to say, "We use state-of-the-art technology," "We have raised our standard of care for our patients," "We use the latest technology for our patients," "We perform oral abnormality screenings on every patient every time." A skilled marketing professional within your practice can translate those commitments into measurable growth.

Most dental professionals have heard a story—perhaps from personal experience or a colleague—of a patient returning to say, "Thank you, you saved my life." That kind of genuine, word-of-mouth marketing is priceless. Patients share those experiences with their friends, family, and neighbors, spreading the message that "my dental office rocks because they found X, Y, Z, which could have killed me if they had not." It raises the standard of care, which is what we are trying to do. This helps bring in new patients to practice, and that is not a metric that shows up on a balance sheet or graph at the end of the month.

Each screening is an opportunity for you to engage with the patient—asking questions and explaining what you are doing and why. Maybe they have risk factors you have identified, and you can educate them on how important screening is given those risks. Cite a few relevant statistics to let them know oral cancer is on the rise and often hard to detect, but that new information and early screening can make a difference. We need to have this conversation with our patients.

Another common excuse for not performing thorough oral abnormality screening is that "it is not covered by insurance." If you can imagine with me, for a moment, that Humana™, or similar healthcare entity covers your automobile. You get into a minor fender bender and need to submit a claim, only to receive an Explanation of Benefits that reads something like this: "We will cover a new engine, but it will be downgraded to a four-cylinder. The bumper will be out of pocket because it is considered cosmetic. This will max out your benefits for the year, so any other repairs will also be out of pocket and must wait."

Education is the key to patient acceptance of any non-covered service, such as screening for their overall health.

Another common reason for not performing an oral abnormality screening is a lack of confidence in one's skill set or knowledge. Only 25% of dentists responding to this survey have attended an oncology or continuing education (CE) course on cancer in the last five years—and a lot has changed in that time. We now have improved diagnostics, a better understanding of causes, and clearer indicators of what to look for. Many clinicians attend CE courses in periodontics, implants, cosmetic dentistry, CAD/CAM and digital impressions, or practice management, but they have not been to one on cancer or oral abnormalities. Again, in the survey I conducted, 17% of respondents could not remember the last time they attended a CE on cancer. Almost 15% said they knew it had been more than three years—and I think 15% is too many.

For those of us who graduated "back in the dark ages," we did not know what we did not know. However, with the advances in diagnostics, technology, and research, there is really no excuse anymore. If you feel you could use a refresher on how to perform an oral abnormality screening, there are many excellent options available to help you feel confident:

- This YouTube video will walk you through the oral care examination step by step: https://www.youtube.com/watch?v=q9kPdQMyU40
- Oral Cancer Consulting has a step-by-step tutorial available: https://oralcancerconsulting.com/cotten-method-guide
- As with other cancers, patients can engage in routine self-exams. There is a site I urge you to check out: https://checkyourmouth.org/wp/I
- The Oral Cancer Foundation has a wealth of information and suggestions to support early detection: https://oralcancerfoundation.org/

Many practitioners are skeptical of adjunct devices. Autofluorescent diagnostic aids assist in discovering potential lesions more effectively when used in conjunction with a physical exam and patient history review—not by replacing them! Autofluorescence technology is not new; it has been in use since the 1990s. It allows practitioners to observe oral abnormalities for changes in tissue density, better delineate lesion boundaries, and obtain reliable photographic documentation. They are simple to use. Simply stating or documenting "lesion is on the right cheek" is not descriptive enough, especially if you are referring the patient to an oral surgeon or ENT specialist. However, you can send the image to the specialist. They will see exactly what you saw and where you saw it, and it allows for checking lesion progression over time.

Certain lesions need to be biopsied. They may come back not cancerous but dysplastic. If they are dysplastic, they need to be followed closely, routinely, and frequently. You also gain documented proof that the screening was performed. It is not difficult and does not take much time. My research also showed that approximately 77% of dental offices do not use an adjunct device. Of those, about 20% reported not using one, citing a lack of evidence for their effectiveness. They also cited cost and insufficient knowledge about the device as additional reasons. Autofluorescence technology comes in many forms, and you need to choose the one that works best for your practice. It becomes an opportunity to elevate your education.

High-Risk Areas and Risk Factors

High-risk areas for possible cancerous lesions include the underside of the tongue and the floor of the mouth. Also risky, but slightly less common, are the lateral tongue surface, the back of the mouth, and the top of the throat. Some risk factors that can be determined during the patient's medical history review are past and present tobacco use, alcohol use, and viral exposure to HPV, HIV, and Epstein-Barr. Chronic cheek or lip chewing, being immunocompromised, and excessive sun exposure are a few others. Many of these risk factors are modifiable and listed on the left of the chart below, while others are not modifiable. We cannot change who we are, our history, or our age.

TABLE 1 Risk Factors for Oral Cancer

Modifiable	Non-modifiable
Tobacco use (smoke, smokeless, electronic)	Family history
Alcohol use	Personal history
Combination of alcohol and tobacco	Age
Sun exposure	Gender
Environmental toxins	Race

High-risk sexual behavior	Immunosuppression

CHAPTER 8

EARLY DETECTION AND THE POWER OF PROTOCOL

Early diagnosis is key to surviving oral cancer. We need to eliminate barriers such as delayed diagnoses, limited access to care, poor service coordination, and lost follow-up. Abnormalities don't automatically translate into an oral cancer diagnosis. Many practitioners believe they have Superman's X-ray vision and can detect cancerous lesions with the naked eye! In fact, general practitioners misdiagnosed over 45% of oral lesions submitted to pathology (Kondori, 2011). They also frequently assumed the patient didn't *look* like they should have cancer because they were young, wealthy, athletic, or held important positions in the community.

HPV and Oral Cancer: The Facts

Approximately 50% of new human papillomavirus (HPV) infections occur among individuals aged 15 to 24 years (oralcancerfoundation.org, 2025)!

- 79 million people are currently living with HPV.
- 14 million people are newly diagnosed each year.
- 7% of individuals between the ages of 14 and 69 have an oral strain of HPV.
- Oral HPV occurs more commonly in men than in women.
- Three out of every five people carry at least one strain of over 200 identified strains of HPV.
- The most prevalent strains of HPV relating to oral cancers are HPV-16 and HPV-18.

The HPV vaccine is recommended beginning at age nine for both boys and girls. Individuals who start the vaccine on or after their 15th birthday require three doses given over six months. Experts have also expanded the recommended age range for vaccination to include adults up to age 40 to help protect against several types of cancers that may develop in midlife.

An infection with even one of the high-risk strains of HPV *does not necessarily mean that oral cancer will develop!* In most cases, the immune system clears the infection before malignancy can occur. The good news is HPV-positive oropharyngeal cancers are biologically different from other head and neck cancers—they are much easier to treat and have better outcomes. The challenge, however, is that HPV-related oral cancers primarily occur in the oropharynx rather than the oral cavity itself, making early detection difficult because these lesions develop too far back in the throat to be easily seen during routine examinations.

Saving Lives with a SNAP

S N A P

The S is for **say** "I'm performing an oral abnormality screening." Educate your patient as to why. Take an intraoral image of the area for reevaluation, to send to referring doctors, and for documentation purposes.

The N is for **never** say, "if it's not better, come back." Schedule an appointment in two weeks to re-evaluate.

The A is for **always** follow up. Benign lesions can evolve into malignancies. It also protects your liability.

If lichen planus is suspected, a biopsy should be indicated during the initial visit to confirm the diagnosis, followed by close monitoring over time for any changes that might indicate malignant transformation. Long-term studies of patients with lichen planus indicate a higher-than-average rate of malignant transformation (Agha-Hossein, 2023).

The P is for **pathologist**. The histologic interpretation of an abnormality demands the specialty expertise of an oral pathologist, not biopsy eyes. Dental superpowers can't determine, just through outward appearances, what's happening at the cellular level (Cotton, 2021).

Emerging Diagnostic Tools

Several studies have found that salivary levels of specific proteins are elevated in whole saliva from patients with oral squamous cell carcinoma (Streckfus et al., 2015). Point-of-care assays are now available that determine if a biomarker is low, moderate, or high risk, allowing for immediate referral for biopsy if results are abnormal. One such test is currently in clinical trials in Europe, with FDA approval expected in the United States in the near future.

Oral brush cytology is another point-of-care option within the dental setting. The kit contains all the necessary materials. A specialized brush is used to scrape epithelial cells from the suspicious area, which are then transferred to a slide and sent to a laboratory. There, the specimen is examined for any dysplasia that may indicate a precancerous or cancerous lesion.

No screening test is 100% accurate, and some cancers may still go undetected, and painless areas may actually be suspect. The gold standard for an oral cancer diagnosis remains tissue biopsy with a pathological assessment.

The average dentist sees three to five patients a day with abnormalities. It is impractical to biopsy everyone, and most abnormalities are benign, with only about 30% being malignant (Cirillo, 2024). It is perfectly acceptable to wait two weeks and reassess when there is reasonable evidence that the lesion is traumatic or otherwise likely to resolve. But waiting longer than that can result in a later-stage diagnosis, which increases your liability and is harder to treat and cure. If you're referring to an oral surgeon who balks at conducting a biopsy for abnormalities you've found, build a new referral network! Do you feel comfortable telling your patient "It's nothing" and assuming full liability if that turns out not to be true later on down the line?

CHAPTER 9

PREHABILITATION PROTOCOL CHECKLIST

The following checklist outlines the essential steps dental providers should complete when preparing a patient for oncology treatment:

1. Schedule the appointment as soon as possible
2. Complete a full, comprehensive clinical examination
3. Assign caries and periodontal risk levels
4. Develop an appropriate treatment plan
5. Create an individualized oral hygiene management plan
6. Consult with the patient's oncologist

1. Schedule the appointment as soon as possible

The front office serves as a critical gateway for patients, and its understanding of prehabilitation concepts, the importance of dental care for oncology patients, and the need for urgency cannot be overstated. The last thing a newly diagnosed cancer patient should hear is that the next available appointment isn't for another six weeks! Long waiting times for dental appointments can derail timely clearance. Extended waiting times can significantly delay dental clearance and jeopardize the timely initiation of cancer treatment. If no urgency is felt by the individual answering the phone or the schedule coordinator, these patients are likely to go elsewhere or ignore the oncologist's recommendation altogether.

This applies to current patients as well as new patient referrals. Scheduling dental treatment needs to be done as quickly as possible, particularly if the patient may require procedures involving nonrestorable teeth or infection control. Dental staff can adjust their schedules. Elective procedures can be moved by calling the patient with a simple explanation— "We have a patient that was recently diagnosed with cancer. Would you be willing to move your appointment to next week?" is often well received. You can advocate for your patients by:

Prioritizing scheduling for newly diagnosed cancer patients. Treating cancer patients as urgent cases—not routine cleanings, assisting them in navigating insurance, referrals, and follow-up care.

The goodwill you build with both patient groups will offset any temporary loss of production. Prehabilitation is urgent, not optional, and front office staff must understand the importance of timely scheduling.

More than 20% of unplanned health care visits from cancer patients stem from a simple need to speak with someone on their care team. Telemedicine is highly effective in many ways and represents the future of reducing unnecessary acute in-office care visits from patients, even those with cancer. Once a patient is established in your practice, telemedicine can be an excellent way to address many concerns as they arise. Dental offices need defined protocols for such communications. The hygienist is ideally positioned to coordinate communication among all of the patients' providers and present those findings to the dental team.

2. Complete a full, comprehensive clinical examination

Beginning with a thorough medical history review is essential—even for *that* patient who insists they don't understand what any of the questions have to do with their teeth. "We have all heard, "Why do you need to know?" "What does that have to do my mouth?" "I'm just getting my teeth cleaned." These moments underscore the ongoing challenge of communicating systemic oral connection. A comprehensive assessment includes an FMX, comprehensive periodontal charting, and identification of conditions that could cause issues during periods of immunosuppression. The evaluation must consist of detailed documentation of:

- Caries risk
- Periodontal status
- Restorative needs
- Presence of implants or prosthetics
- Documentation of potential sources of gingival trauma
- Oral abnormality screening

This baseline data will enable you to evaluate the effectiveness of product recommendations and guide treatment decisions.

3. Assign caries and periodontal risk levels

Assign risk levels based on a patient's current oral health status, their dental and medical history, any high-risk habits (e.g., smoking, alcohol consumption), relevant comorbidities (e.g., diabetes, heart disease), and their overall level of commitment to care. This process should follow a recognized framework, such as the CAMBRA® protocol (https://dentistry.ucsf.edu/research/cambra). Incorporate point-of-care salivary diagnostics, including salivary flow rate, pH testing, and periodontal pathogen analysis. A thorough risk assessment guides personalized care.

4. Develop an appropriate treatment plan

Address all restorative needs promptly and fabricate custom trays. Address nonrestorable teeth and active infections first. Allow at least 14 days for healing before starting oncology treatment. Any required crowns, fillings, periodontal therapy, or the removal of orthodontic attachments, such as aligner buttons, bands, brackets, and even fixed retainers, should be considered emergent care, especially in a patient with a head and neck cancer. Taking impressions or scans for custom trays also needs to be done early on in treatment. Trays can be fabricated later when they are required for medicaments (fluoride, remineralization, desensitization, etc.). Obtaining impressions later may not be possible once the patient begins experiencing mucositis and mouth inflammation. If there isn't enough time to complete all restorative treatment before oncology treatment begins, consider using silver diamine fluoride for its stabilizing effect. It is not always pretty, but it will arrest decay until restorative care can be completed.

5. Create an individualized oral hygiene management plan

This phase also includes developing a plan for decreasing the patient's bacterial load. Cancer therapy alters the oral and intestinal microflora, increasing the risk of infection and inflammation. Cancer-therapy–

induced oral mucositis often coincides with periodontal-based bacteria (particularly P. gingivalis), which further inhibits wound healing. Patients should receive clear education on what to expect and things to watch for during their treatment.

Stress the importance of meticulous oral hygiene and increase the frequency of recare visits to support early detection of decay, address sensitivity, reduce bacterial load, and reinforce the preventive and educational phases of prehabilitation concepts. Provide patients with sensitive, deep clean, or postsurgical brushes. Power toothbrushes are great but may not be tolerated well or even advisable for a cancer patient in current treatment.

Interdental cleaning is essential! If patients have never flossed, the start of cancer treatment is probably not the time to start! However, we still need to reduce the bacterial load, which means interdental cleaning is necessary.

Patients can use a water flosser on a very low setting and gradually increase the intensity as their tolerance allows, or they can use quality interdental brushes as a gentler alternative. Many oncology teams tell patients not to floss at all. And while there may be occasions where this makes sense, for the most part, it underscores a gap in understanding within the medical community about what we do and why we do it. This presents an opportunity for us to educate both patients and medical colleagues about oral biofilm dynamics and the risk of bacteremia. The risk of bacteremia from interdental cleaning is no greater than the risk produced by regular chewing.

From a nutritional standpoint, introduce 100% xylitol into the patient's daily regimen. Encourage consistent use of 100% xylitol-sweetened products, as they neutralize oral pH, inhibit bacterial growth, stimulate saliva, satisfy sweet cravings, and help keep blood glucose levels stable. Xylitol products are available in many forms, including pastes, rinses, sprays, gum, and mints. Their regular use will improve treatment outcomes. Keep in mind that certain flavors may not be tolerated, such as strong mint or cinnamon. Patients should also be advised to avoid sharp, crunchy, hot, spicy, and highly acidic foods, as well as alcohol.

Cancer treatments can significantly affect a patient's ability to swallow and greatly alter taste, smell, and overall sensory perception of food. Sensory tolerance, particularly to certain textures, is often heightened in cancer patients, and what they can comfortably tolerate will vary throughout their treatment. Many patients will experience altered smell and taste, leading to a loss of interest in food or the common complaint that "everything tastes like dirt." Traditionally recommended nutritional supplements are incredibly high in sugar. Ensure® comes in a version with only 1 gram of sugar. Certain therapy medications increase cravings for high sugar foods and carbohydrates, so be sure your patients are aware of the sugar content of what they consume and that there are other options.

Patients should also be counseled on using sugar-free lozenges and candies to relieve xerostomia. Constantly sipping water to deal with dry mouth should be avoided. Drinking water with meals and to hydrate is fine and essential but continually sipping water throughout the day can be counterproductive to hydrating the oral tissues and balancing the oral flora. This is covered more in the book *Get Your Spit Together! Your Saliva May Hold the Secret to Better*

Dental Checkups, 2022. Oral hygiene management is essential for healing and comfort, while education enhances care coordination, and nutritional guidance supports systemic and oral health.

6. Consult with the patient's oncologist

One of the most critical steps in the prehabilitation protocol checklist is scheduling a consultation with the patient's oncologist and care team. It is an opportunity to educate the oncology team on dental topics, such as the fact that a "prophy" is more than just a polish and can be invasive depending on the patient's periodontal health. If nonsurgical periodontal therapy is needed, educate the oncologist and care team on how reducing bacterial load in the mouth can positively affect the outcomes of cancer treatments. If the patient needs any dental treatment—even treatment that is usually considered routine—it becomes not so "routine" for cancer patients. Share research on prehabilitation and oral–systemic links.

You can contact the patient's oncology office to schedule a meeting to introduce yourself and the practice and explain that you have a mutual patient who has shared their diagnosis with you (Vega & Bernard, 2016). The following is an example of an outreach message:

We will support Ms. Smith's oral health needs throughout her treatment. If you or Ms. Smith have any concerns about her oral health—or if any of your other patients need a dental home—please feel free to reach out. We are here to help. Our goal is to prevent, or at least minimize, any oral side effects of treatment that may impact on their quality of life. Please also let us know your preferred communication method, whether fax, email, phone, or virtual meetings—so we can coordinate with your team as smoothly as possible.

Treatment Coordination

Dental treatment during cancer therapy must be coordinated around Nadir, making it essential to understand the patient's treatment cycle and cocktail regimen. Having a strong working relationship with the oncology team enables timely communication and safe scheduling. Prophylactic antibiotics are still routinely recommended for oncology patients. But again, when in doubt, check with the oncologist. Always coordinate with the oncology team!

Nadir (pronounced *nay-duhr*) is an important consideration when planning dental treatment during cancer treatment. Derived from Latin for "the lowest point," the term refers to the period when blood cell counts—particularly neutrophils—are at their lowest. This low point usually occurs 10–14 days after an infusion. Coordinate dental care around the patient's lowest immune point and always clarify with the oncology team whether prophylactic antibiotics are needed for planned procedures.

Leukopenia refers to the drop in white blood cell levels that occurs following chemotherapy infusion. During this period, patients are at an increased risk of infection, septicemia, and bleeding.

Neutropenia refers to a neutrophil count lower than 500. Neutrophils are a type of white blood cell that helps the body fight off bacterial infections. During the neutropenic nadir, patients are more likely to contract infections, especially given the inflammatory nature of periodontal disease and its destruction of connective tissue (Vanhoecke et al., 2015).

Thrombocytopenia refers to a decrease in platelet count, which can cause clotting issues and an increased risk of bleeding.

Anemia refers to a decrease in red blood cells, which can affect tissue function.

The patient's risk for dental treatment is determined using a CBC and a PT/INR, both of which are routinely performed during oncology visits. It is essential to obtain them before any dental treatment begins. This underscores the importance of maintaining a strong relationship with the oncology team to ensure you can get those test results. There are guidelines available to help determine when and when not to provide dental treatment based on test results (Cotter, 2019).

Important Blood Values for Immunosuppressed Patients Undergoing Invasive Dental Procedures

Test	Value Range	Recommendation
ANC (Neutrophils)	> 2.0 (2,000/mm³)	No antibiotic prophylaxis
ANC (Neutrophils)	1.0 – 2.0 (1,000 - 2,000/mm³)	Antibiotic prophylaxis according to AHA guidelines
ANC (Neutrophils)	< 1.0 (1,000/mm³)	Refer to dental oncologist or oral surgeon
Platelets	>75,000	No platelet support therapy
Platelets	50,000 - 75,000	Local hemostasis such as pressure, microfibrillar, and sutures
Platelets	<50,000	Platelet transfusion one hour prior to procedure

There are guidelines for the PT/INR results, too. See Table 3 below.

Table 3 PT/INR Guidelines

Cancer patients are at increased risk of stroke, seizures, DVT's and pulmonary embolisms. As a result, their treatment often involves being placed on blood thinners. This is why it is important to have recent readings and consult with the oncologist prior to dental treatment including routine prophylaxis on a healthy mouth.

INR RATES	
NORMAL	1.0
ACCEPTABLE RANGE	2.0 – 3.0
RISK OF EXCESSIVE BLEEDING	3.0 ↑

Clinical Considerations

Once laboratory values have been obtained and the patient is cleared for scheduling, several special considerations need to be kept in mind. Morning appointments are generally preferred, as patients tend to tire throughout the day. A patient with anemia may tend to be lethargic, irritable, and forgetful, requiring precise written home care instructions. Many times, the patient is cold even in the middle of summer, so keeping a blanket on hand is advised.

Radiotherapy Effects and Positioning Challenges

A common long-term effect of head and neck radiotherapy is blocked carotid arteries. Patients may also experience baroreceptor damage, which impairs blood pressure regulation. Even if a patient's blood pressure is normal at the start of an appointment, it can suddenly increase or decrease, leading to syncope.

Positioning the head during dental cleaning, radiographs, or examinations can restrict blood flow to the brain, increasing the risk of syncope from vascular occlusion. Head and neck cancer patients experience chronic fatigue of the neck muscles, making it difficult for them to keep their head upright or move backward. These patients often experience degeneration of cervical vertebrae, which can make certain positions painful. Recommending warm, moist heat before and after appointments and/or the use of anti-inflammatory medications when appropriate is helpful for jaw and neck pain.

Head and neck cancer patients need to increase the vertical dimension. Trismus is unpredictable in both frequency and severity. Specific exercises can help with this, which is why having specialized support from an orthomyofunctional therapist is helpful.

Local Anesthetic Considerations

The use of local anesthetics containing vasoconstrictors in cancer patients is considered controversial, as it may increase the risk of adverse cardiovascular events. A comparative study by Laragnoit et al is the first to examine the use of lidocaine with and without epinephrine in patients with a history of heart failure. A total of 72 patients scheduled for tooth extraction and restoration procedures were randomly assigned to receive lidocaine with or without epinephrine.

According to the study, systolic and diastolic blood pressure increased significantly in both groups during the procedure, while maximum heart rate declined. However, there were no differences in blood pressure, heart rate, or arrhythmias between the two groups, although patients who did not receive epinephrine reported significantly higher pain levels (Laragnoit, 2018).

The possible presence of vascular blockage and irregular blood pressure readings means patients must be closely monitored during dental treatment for signs of a transient ischemic attack (TIA) (Plummer et al., 2011). Sudden dizziness, slurred speech, weakness, or numbness may all signal a possible TIA.

- A structured protocol ensures safe, timely, and effective care.
- Early intervention prevents complications and improves outcomes.
- Communication with oncology teams is essential.
- Every detail—from appointment timing to toothbrush softness—can make a difference.
- Prehabilitation is a team effort—and you're a vital part of it.

CHAPTER 10

PRODUCTS AND PERSONALIZATION IN CANCER CARE

There is no single one-size-fits-all product! Patients should be offered *choices*, not just instructions, because no individual product can meet every need. If a patient dislikes a product and is not using it, it's not doing anybody any good. The product must be palatable and contain appropriate, well-tolerated ingredients. Some products contain too much sodium or citric acid for patients. The key message here is: no universal product works for everyone!

"I always ask, 'How's that working for you?' If they shrug or say 'meh,' it's time to switch."

Start with the Right Questions

The first questions you should be asking a patient when they present with oral symptoms from their cancer therapy are:

- What is the desired outcome?
- Is it to provide moisture?

- Is it to provide pain relief?
- Is it to provide wound healing?
- Is it to prevent decay?

Additional questions to discuss with the patient when selecting products include:

- Is the product best suited for daytime use, overnight use, or both?
- When are symptoms most severe—morning, afternoon, or evening?
- What is the patient's profession? Do they speak frequently in roles such as sales, teaching, or customer service? Or do they work in positions with minimal verbal interaction, such as software development, data entry, or auto repair?
- How often can the product be used safely? Do the instructions limit use to three times per day, or can it be applied as needed?

Adapt to Changing Needs

Patients have to be able to use the product. What works great for one person may not work for someone else. What worked for a patient today may not work for them next month. As they go through cancer treatment, their needs are going to change, so having a variety of products for them to choose from is preferred. No two cancer patients are alike—and neither are their oral care needs. As dental professionals, we must be equipped with a flexible, evidence-based toolkit that adapts to each patient's symptoms, preferences, and treatment stage.

Recommended Products and Tools

Sensitive deep-clean or postsurgical brushes, such as those available from Curaprox® or TePe®, are great recommendations and are superior to your average "soft" toothbrushes found on store shelves. Ideally, clinicians should keep a supply of these brushes in the office to offer to patients who require them.

A toothbrush harbors more than 100 million bacteria, including *E. coli* and *Staphylococcus*. For this reason, it is recommended that toothbrushes be replaced monthly or after any infection. Frequent sanitizing is also essential, especially when bleeding is present, and covering the toothbrush when not in use helps reduce exposure to aerosolized bacteria in the environment (InteliDent®).

Additional support products can also be beneficial. Using a product like Steraligner® for appliance and tray care will eliminate 99% of the 17 most common bacteria, yeast, and mold found on oral appliances with just a 3-minute soak. Steraligner® will also sanitize a toothbrush in under 1 minute.

Many oncology teams advise against flossing; use this as an opportunity to educate them about biofilm and the risk of bacteremia. As previously mentioned, if a patient has never flossed, now is not the time to start. The concern about introducing bacteremia while the patient is immuno-compromised is valid. However, leaving significant amounts of bacteria and debris in the mouth can cause inflammation, which ultimately increases the risk. Chewing is just as likely to cause bacteremia as flossing. Supportive alternatives could include introducing patients to water flossers used on a very low setting and/or quality-sensitive interdental brushes (Curaprox® or TePe®), along with education on their proper use (Jolkovsky & Lyle, 2015).

Product Selection and Patient-Centered Care

Suppose there is a need to reduce bacterial load in the mouth. In that case, products such as StellaLife® and PerioScience® contain natural ingredients, accelerate wound healing due to their bacteria-fighting qualities, don't stain teeth, and hydrate the mucosa. An adjunct to consider is the use of oral care probiotics, such as BioGaia® or ProBiora®, to reduce bacterial load and restore a more balanced oral flora.

Does the patient have any salivary flow, or is it significantly reduced? When salivary flow is absent, artificial saliva substitutes such as SalivaMax® or NeutraSal® are appropriate. These products are primarily palliative, providing symptomatic relief when salivary function is lost due to damage to the salivary glands. It is essential to note that some products have multiple side effects that may not be acceptable for certain patients (Salum et al., 2018).

If the patient does have some salivary function, some products stimulate salivary flow while also supporting saliva's protective properties. A recent review comparing different artificial saliva products found that all tested products reduced signs and symptoms of xerostomia, with some herbal products showing greater improvement in cases of radiation-induced xerostomia. But because each product had advantages, worked better in some sites than others, and offered different durations of relief, it was challenging to identify a single product that stood out (Assery, 2019).

Hopefully, you have performed pH testing to determine if the patient's oral environment is acidic. It is essential to investigate the inherent pH of the products we recommend and that patients may end up using. There are multiple ways to perform these tests, ranging from simple, low-cost test strips from Amazon® to more sophisticated tests sent to a lab for analysis for a fee (Oral DNA®). Patients appreciate visual confirmation of whether their efforts are practical. Testing also provides needed documentation that an assessment has been performed, resulting in a diagnosis and a need for a particular treatment. If a patient is using a product for dry mouth or any other oral condition and it is working for them, we don't necessarily want to discontinue its use. But if the product itself has an acidic pH, we would need to buffer the environment with a product like Basic Bites®, which provides a healthy pH balance and is enamel-enriching.

Early in treatment, scans or impressions should have been taken to make custom trays for fluoride and remineralization therapies. Both Remin Pro® and MI Paste® help with hypersensitivity, remineralization, and caries prevention. MI paste® is contraindicated for those with a true milk protein allergy, which is different than lactose intolerance. It is a two-in-one product with fluoride and ACP. Remin Pro® does not carry this restriction and can be used in patients who cannot tolerate milk-derived proteins.

In-office fluoride varnishes need to be applied frequently (three to four times a year). Toothpaste delivery is the most common form of at-home fluoride treatment, but compliance with the ideal application process can sometimes be a problem with some individuals. Prescription-strength fluoride is available in gel form (Gel-Kam® or PreviDent®) for use in custom trays, which might be an acceptable alternative for patients.

When recommending products for oral hygiene at home or for symptom relief, it's not about a product being right or wrong, good or bad—it's about offering patients choices. Symptoms will vary widely from patient to patient, depending on the underlying causes and the specific treatments they are receiving, and these symptoms may also change over time. Xerostomia, for example, is very transient and affected by many factors. Proper treatment often involves multiple therapies.

Education and Delivery Matter

If you hand patients a bag of products, they are likely to set it aside or forget about it entirely—and may even wonder, "What am I supposed to do with these again?" Go slowly and find their individual needs. Don't just dump a stack of literature or products on them. A good resource for recommended products is Side Effect Support: https://sideeffectsupport.com/.

Providing patients with education about what to expect regarding their dental needs, the events they should be aware of during treatment, and offering resources available to them are key components of the Prehabilitation Protocol. This includes guidance such as: "If this happens, call your oncologist," "When this happens, try this product," "If this happens, call us and let us know." Having a consultation with the patient's oncologist is critical. You need to establish a relationship with them to guide the patient through their treatment to achieve healthy dentition. Remember:

1. Go Slow
    - Don’t overwhelm patients with too much at once.
    - Provide written and verbal instructions.
    - Tailor kits and recommendations to their current symptoms.

2. Be Specific
    - “Use this rinse after meals and before bed.”
    - “Avoid cinnamon and mint if your mouth feels raw.”

3. Offer Support
    - Give your number or email if appropriate.

- Encourage them to call with questions or changes in symptoms.

- ❖ No single product works for every patient.
- ❖ Ask questions to guide product selection
- ❖ The right product is the one the patient will use.
- ❖ Symptoms evolve and so should your recommendations.
- ❖ Education is just as important as the tools themselves.
- ❖ Stock high-quality tools and offer choices—not just instructions.
- ❖ Your guidance can dramatically improve comfort, compliance, and outcomes.

CHAPTER 11

SURVIVORSHIP AND EMOTIONAL SUPPORT FROM A DENTAL PRACTICE

Cancer doesn't end when treatment does. Survivors and their families often face a long, uncertain road filled with physical, emotional, and psychological challenges. As dental professionals, we are uniquely positioned to walk that road with them—not just as clinicians, but as trusted advocates. Every day in our offices, we have patients undergoing medical treatment or their caregivers, which gives us a unique opportunity to make a difference.

We can make a difference by educating caregivers, other providers, co-hygienists, oncology nurses, oncology departments, and endorsing referrals to those with expertise. We can offer ourselves as a resource to patients as they progress through their treatment and questions or needs arise. This is part of the compassion that led us to this profession and lets us make a positive impact on an individual's quality of life. Treating a patient in your office or the family member of one who has received a cancer diagnosis is to remember that cancer is not over when the treatment is over. It will affect everyone close to them.

Recognizing Emotional Distress

You may be the first person to notice signs of depression, post-traumatic stress disorder (PTSD), survivor's guilt, or caregiver burnout. Four features characterize PTSD:

1. An unexpected event. Who expects to hear the words "You have cancer"?
2. An overwhelming event. Depending on the diagnosis, those words can be mind-boggling and potentially devastating.
3. The individual was unprepared or unable to cope with the event. Many go into denial and wrestle with the cancer diagnosis.
4. A feeling of helplessness to prevent or change the event. How often do you hear about an individual who never smoked, was physically fit, ate healthy, and was still diagnosed with cancer (Cameron, 2015)?

PTSD in a cancer patient can be the direct result of a traumatic event or of an aspect of prior care, like noticing symptoms or going for a scan. Every new lump, bump, or pain creates anxiety. Even though I am 10 years out of my own diagnosis, I still experience this.

Panic Attacks versus Anxiety Attacks

Panic attacks occur suddenly, unexpectedly, and typically only last for a few minutes, whereas anxiety attacks can persist for months. Either can arise in specific situations, such as before a medical procedure or in a dental office, though panic attacks often occur without an identifiable trigger. Patients may experience a strong urge to escape the situation, even when there is no immediate physical threat.

I have witnessed this with patients in my chair: sometimes the patient who is being "difficult" in the office is experiencing extreme anxiety. Panic attacks can be very alarming and may include symptoms such as shortness of breath, a racing heartbeat, dizziness, sweating, shaking, chest pain, choking feelings, and overwhelming fear, which are often confused with symptoms of a heart attack. These intense feelings may be constant or come and go. Some pass with time, while others last longer. Patients might feel like they're on an emotional roller-coaster. There is no right or wrong way for a patient to feel. You can treat a patient, and everything's going fine, and then suddenly, *boom!* Anxiety can manifest in a crying jag that the patient is unable to control or in irritability and unexpected anger, and cancer survivors don't always have control over their emotions. Many start crying for no reason and become irritable, going from zero to 60 in no time flat.

"Sometimes the 'difficult' patient is actually just terrified."

How Dental Professionals Can Respond

The following strategies can help dental professionals respond appropriately and compassionately to patients experiencing emotional distress:

- Practice active listening – Let them talk. Don't rush to fix things.

- Respect their boundaries – Some want to talk. Others don't.
- Avoid platitudes – "You'll be fine" can feel dismissive.
- Be patient and empathetic.
- Recognize emotional triggers.
- Offer reassurance and flexibility.
- Document emotional responses and follow-up need.
- Refer to mental health professionals when appropriate.

Managing Panic and Anxiety in the Dental Office

If you find yourself dealing with a patient experiencing panic or anxiety attack in the office, there are grounding techniques you can help them use, like the 5-4-3-2-1 sensory method or the 5-5-5 breathing method.

The 5-4-3-2-1 sensory method begins by asking the patient to name five things they see, four things they feel, three things they hear, two things they smell, and one thing they taste. This often is enough to help calm a patient. During a panic attack, these sensations may be intense, but they typically peak and pass within a few minutes.

The 5-5-5 breathing method involves asking the patient to breathe in for 5 seconds, hold their breath for 5 seconds, and then breathe out for 5 seconds. You can continue with this sequence until their thoughts slow down, or you notice they are starting to experience some relief.

Be consistent. Your presence and reliability matter. Some reassuring phrases you can use include:

- "You're safe here."
- "Let's take a moment."
- "Would you like to pause or continue?"

Survivor's guilt is often considered a serious symptom of PTSD and a heavy burden. Patients may ask themselves:

- "Why did I survive when others didn't?"
- "What more could I have done?"
- "Do I deserve to be happy?"

Research estimates that as many as 90% of people who live through events where others died or suffered experience feelings of guilt (Cheney, 2025). This is part of the healing process and is normal after surviving a physically or emotionally traumatic event. As health care providers, our role is not to fix their cancer diagnosis, but to acknowledge it, validate it, and offer them our support as they walk the road of healing, realizing that there are parts of the journey that must be walked alone. Respect their need for privacy. There are no quick and easy fixes.

CHAPTER 12

COMPASSIONATE CARE: PALLIATIVE VS HOSPICE

Let's talk about the difference between palliative care and hospice care. Palliative care takes place in the hospital, whereas hospice care can be wherever the patient calls home and can be at any stage of the disease. Hospice is initiated when doctors predict that the patient has six months or less to live. Palliative care can be covered by insurance or self-pay, and palliative care patients do not have to meet the exact eligibility requirements as hospice care patients. While the objective of both hospice and palliative care is pain and symptom relief, the prognosis and goals of care tend to be different.

Palliative care is comfort care with or without curative intent. In contrast, hospice care is comfort care without curative intent. It is typically chosen when the patient no longer has curative options or decides not to pursue treatment because the side effects outweigh the benefits.

Palliative care, also referred to as comfort care, is specialized medical care for people living with a serious illness, focused on relieving symptoms and stress. In a palliative care program, patients can opt for extensive life-prolonging treatment since the treatment routines will be adhered to by medical providers. There is no limit on when a patient should receive this type of care; it works well for patients seeking comfort at any stage of illness, whether chronic or terminal. The goal is to improve the quality of life for both the patient and their family.

Palliative care is based on the patient's needs, not on their prognosis. It is appropriate at any age and at any stage of a serious illness and can be provided alongside curative or life-prolonging treatment. Palliative care does not mean death. Palliative care includes managing the physical symptoms, pain, and ongoing treatments. It includes providing emotional and spiritual support, support with daily tasks and personal hygiene, extending support to family and friends, and assisting in preparing plans for advanced care.

Some of the serious illnesses that receive palliative care are:

- Heart problems
- Cancer
- Chronic respiratory illnesses

- Acquired immune deficiency syndrome
- Diabetes
- Chronic kidney and liver disease
- Multiple sclerosis
- Rheumatoid arthritis
- Chronic congenital disabilities
- Neurological disorders

You may know someone or have seen advertisements for medications that are described as a "once a month injection" or medication for conditions such as multiple sclerosis, rheumatoid arthritis, or Parkinson's. These types of medications are considered palliative care. Studies show that patients live longer and better with palliative care because of its focus on quality of life. In addition, palliative care can help patients better understand their treatment options. Palliative care provides that extra layer of support in addition to everything the person already has in place, such as chemotherapy, radiation, physical or occupational therapy, or planned surgery. This care can be pursued at the time of diagnosis, during active curative treatment, follow-ups, and at the end of life. As dental providers, we play a significant role in this.

As a dental provider, you may be called upon to visit patients in hospice at the hospital or at their home. If you provide oral hygiene instructions to your hospice patient, you can bill "behavior management by report." This will require a narrative, such as:

> "Oncology-induced hyposalivation, fungal overgrowth, and multiple medications. I spent 15 minutes with a caregiver teaching oral hygiene techniques for comfort and oral health."

Hospice care is comfort care without curative intent. End-of-life or hospice care programs are provided wherever the patient calls home and under the supervision of hospice professionals. Hospice mainly relies on the caregiver and the nurse administering the hospice care. The team comprises end-of-life care specialists, doctors, nurses, volunteers, aides, grief counselors, social workers, nutritionists, and chaplains.

Hospice is indicated when:

1. The patient has limited ability to care for themselves.
2. The patient has received curative treatment but is no longer benefiting from it.
3. The patient does not qualify for an appropriate clinical trial.
4. There is no evidence that further treatment would be effective.
5. The patient is stable, allowing the care team to develop the plan of care and implement it.
6. The patient becomes less stable, and the plan of care is adjusted to begin to prepare the patient emotionally for what lies ahead.
7. The patient's condition deteriorates, shifting priority to end-of-life care. As the patient nears the end of life, the focus shifts to managing symptoms and providing emotional and spiritual support. After the patient dies, hospice addresses the emotional and spiritual pain

suffered by loved ones for a period of time, sometimes over 12 months.

Respecting the Patient's Journey

There are three Cs of hospice: commitment, conviction, and compassion. When visiting with an individual diagnosed with a serious or terminal disease, think before you speak. Avoid saying, "Don't worry, you'll be fine," and instead say, "I'm really sorry" or "I hope it will be okay." Don't refer to their cancer as "the good cancer." These statements downplay what they are going through. Try not to be overly grave and mournful. "I know someone who had the same thing as you" (no two cancers are the same). If you know someone with the same type of cancer as your patient, offer to connect the two of them. Never tell stories with unhappy endings and refrain from physical assessments. Comments about how they look, especially negative ones, are not helpful. They don't need changes in their weight or hair loss pointed out to them. One comment can instantly undo someone's upbeat mood. Follow their lead. Let the person with cancer set the tone about what they want to talk about. It doesn't always have to be about cancer. Chances are, they want to feel as normal as possible. Tell them about something funny that happened. Allow them to talk about cancer if they want. Save the puppy dog eyes and voice.

"You don't have to have all the answers—just a sympathetic ear."

Your role as a dental professional when your patient is in hospice is to provide oral hygiene guidance to support their comfort and to be available for home visits, if appropriate.

- Advocacy is about presence, persistence, and compassion.
- You are more than a provider—you are a lifeline.
- Your support can change the course of a patient's journey.
- Never underestimate the power of listening, following up, and showing up.

CHAPTER 13

CARRYING THE TORCH

This book began with a promise—to Misty, to my patients, and to every dental professional who wants to do more than pat their patient's arm and offer condolences. It was born from grief, shaped by experience, and fueled by a deep belief that we can do better.

I've walked this road as a caregiver, a clinician, and a survivor. I've seen the pain that cancer inflicts—not just on the body, but on the spirit. And I've seen how a compassionate, informed dental professional can make a difference that ripples far beyond the operatory.

Why This Book Matters

In these pages, I wanted to share ideas, protocols, and perspectives to help you support your patients who are going through or are survivors of cancer. We can be a source of information, guidance, and advice for patients or their family members we see in the office. We are competent providers who can advise, direct, and offer solutions for a wide range of issues. We can also have on hand referrals and other tools to guide them to resources with more information and assistance for matters outside our scope and expertise. Because we develop such a close relationship with our patients, they often see us more frequently than their primary care doctors. Over the years, patients have sometimes even felt more comfortable with us than with their primary care doctors. This presents an opportunity to assess the patient for signs and symptoms of PTSD or depression and possibly intervene if it is appropriate (Manne et al., 2008). Offering information on providers you know within the practice or others in your tribe that offer healing therapies can also be very helpful during this time.

- Oral care is not a luxury, it's a lifeline.
- Prehabilitation is not a buzzword, it's a game-changer.
- Intercollaboration is not optional, it's essential.
- Your role as a dental professional is not small, it's sacred.

I still miss Misty. I think about her almost every day. She wasn't just my best friend—she was my inspiration.

She's the reason I wrote this book, the reason I teach, and the reason I believe so fiercely in this mission.

She didn't get to see her daughter graduate from nursing school. She'll never hold her grandchildren. But her story lives on in every lecture, every article, and every page of this book.

You are not *just* a hygienist or *just* a dentist. You are a trusted voice, a steady hand, and sometimes, the only person who sees the whole patient—not just the diagnosis.

Your Next Steps

1. Start the conversation—with your team, your patients, your local oncology offices.
2. Build your referral network.
3. Create a prehabilitation protocol in your practice.
4. Educate yourself and others.
5. Be the advocate your patients didn't know they needed.

Final Thoughts

To every dental professional reading this: you have the power to change lives. Not with magic. Not with miracles. But with knowledge, compassion, and the courage to care deeply.

Let's raise the standard. Let's close the gap. Let's carry the torch—for Misty, for your patients, and for every life we have the privilege to touch.

REFERENCES

Agha-Hosseini F, Moosavi MS, Ghaffarpour M. Investigating the factors proposed in oral lichen planus malignant transformation: A literature review. Health Sci Rep. 2023 May 17;6(5):e1267. doi: 10.1002/hsr2.1267. PMID: 37205932; PMCID: PMC10189866.

https://www.amenclinics.com/blog/understanding-the-relationship-between-survivors-guilt-and-ptsd/

American Cancer Society medical and editorial content team. (July 2022) American Society of Clinical Oncology (ASCO). Retrieved from https://www.cancer.org/cancer/survivorship/long-term-health-concerns/post-traumatic-stress-disorder-and-cancer.html

Assery, M. K. (2019). Efficacy of artificial salivary substitutes in treatment of xerostomia: a systematic review. Journal of Pharmacy and Bioallied Sciences, 11(Suppl 1), S1-S12.

Atchison, K, Rozier, R, Weintraub, J. 2018 Integration of Oral Health and Primary Care: Communication and Referral. National Academy of Medicine https://nam.edu/perspectives/integration-of-oral-health-and-primary-care-communication-coordination-and-referral/

Bainbridge D, Seow H, Sussman J, Pond G, Martelli-Reid L, Herbert C, Evans W. Multidisciplinary health care professionals' perceptions of the use and utility of a symptom assessment system for oncology patients. J Oncol Pract. 2011 Jan;7(1):19-23. https://ascopubs.org/doi/10.1200/JOP.2010.000015 PMID: 21532805; PMCID: PMC3014504.

Cheney, T. (2025). From Malibu: The Dangers of Survivor's Guilt
Personal Perspective: Facing a natural disaster is traumatic, whatever the outcome. Psychology Today https://www.psychologytoday.com/us/blog/the-bipolar-lens/202501/from-malibu-the-dangers-of-survivors-guilt

Cirillo, N. (2024). Precursor Lesions, Overdiagnosis, and Oral Cancer: A Critical Review. Cancers, 16(8), 1550. https://doi.org/10.3390/cancers16081550

Cotter,J, Dilliard, J What do Lab Values Mean? Dimensions of Dental Hygiene. March 2019;17(3):37–40

Cotton, Susan, Oral Cancer Consulting. *https://oralcancerconsulting.com/*

Czerninski R, Lederman D, Ephros H, and Kerr R. 24 January 2008. Retrieved from https://maaom.memberclicks.net/index.php?option=com_content&view=article&id=138:premalignant-oral-lesions&catid=22:patient-condition-information&Itemid=120

Estilo CL, Van Poznak CH, Wiliams T, Bohle GC, Lwin PT, Zhou Q, Riedel ER, Carlson DL, Schoder H, Farooki A, Fornier M, Halpern JL, Tunick SJ, Huryn JM. Osteonecrosis of the maxilla and mandible in patients with advanced cancer treated with bisphosphonate therapy. Oncologist. 2008 Aug;13(8):911-20. doi: 10.1634/theoncologist.2008-0091. Epub 2008 Aug 11. PMID: 18695259.

Falvo, Joe. (June 27, 2017). Retrieved from https://www.dmdtoday.com/news/professional-

referrals-between-primary-care-physicians-and-dentists

https://familycaregiversonline.net/caregivers-and-addiction/

Grassi L, Spiegel D, Riba M. Advancing psychosocial care in cancer patients. F1000Research. 2017:6. doi: 10.12688/f1000research.11902.1.

Gregoriou PL, Charalambous A, Rousou E, Papastavrou E, Merkouris A. Attitudes of Physicians and Nurses Toward Interprofessional Collaboration: A Systematic Literature Review. Mater Sociomed. 2025;37(1):64-73. doi: 10.5455/msm.2025.37.64-73. PMID: 40098756; PMCID: PMC11910901.

Gubar, Susan. (2018) Retrieved from https://www.nytimes.com/2018/11/15/well/live/tackling-cancer-anxiety.html

Handley NR, Schuchter LM, Bekelman JE. Best practices for reducing unplanned acute care for patients with cancer. J Oncol Pract. 2018;14(5):306-313.

https://ascopubs.org/doi/full/10.1200/JOP.17.0008 1. Accessed April 26, 2018.

Harrison, Pam, Barclay, Laurie MD. Can Marijuana Use Ease Pain/Anxiety in Head and Neck Cancer? Medscape News CME 10/5/2018. https://www.medscape.org/viewarticle/902687

*Hasan, A., Alraisi, S. MRONJ and COVID-19 caution. Br Dent J **230,** 59–60 (2021). https://doi.org/10.1038/s41415-021-2616-9*

M Ishimaru, H Matsui, S Ono, Y Hagiwara, K Morita, H Yasunaga, Preoperative oral care and effect on postoperative complications after major cancer surgery. British Journal of Surgery. 2018;105(12): 1688-1696. doi.org/10.1002/bjs.10915

Islas-Granillo, H., Borges-Yanez, A., Fernandez-Barrera, M. et al. Relationship of hyposalivation and xerostomia in Mexican elderly with socioeconomic, sociodemographic and dental factors. Sci Rep 7, 40686 (2017). doi.org/10.1038/srep40686

Jolkovsky DL, Lyle DM. Safety of a water flosser: a literature review. Compend Contin Educ Dent. 2015 Feb;36(2):146-9. PMID: 25822642..

Kondori I, Mottin RW, Laskin DM. Accuracy of dentists in the clinical diagnosis of oral lesions. Quintessence Int. 2011 Jul-Aug;42(7):575-7. PMID: 21716985.

Laragnoit AB, Neves RS, Neves IL, Vieira JE. Locoregional anesthesia for dental treatment in cardiac patients: a comparative study of 2% plain lidocaine and 2% lidocaine with epinephrine (1:100,000). Clinics (Sao Paulo). 2009;64(3):177-82. doi: 10.1590/s1807-59322009000300005. PMID: 19330241; PMCID: PMC2666461.

Laheij, Alexa & Soet, Johnannes. (2014). Can the oral microflora affect oral ulcerative mucositis?. Current opinion in supportive and palliative care. 8. 10.1097/SPC.0000000000000053.

Manne SL, Winkel G, Rubin S, Edelson M, Rosenblum N, Bergman C, Hernandez E, Carlson J, Rocereto T. Mediators of a coping and communication-enhancing intervention and a supportive counseling intervention among women diagnosed with gynecological cancers. J Consult Clin Psychol. 2008 Dec;76(6):1034-45. doi:10.1037/a0014071. PMID: 19045971; PMCID: PMC2710766.

Mayo Clinic Staff. (2004). Retrieved from https://www.mayoclinic.org/diseases-conditions/cancer/in-depth/mouth-sores/art-20045486

Mayo, Lisa. (2017) Lecture [It's Time to Talk About Sex in Dentistry...HPV and It's Relation to Cancer].

https://www.mskcc.org/news/answers-faq-about-chemotherapy-induced-peripheral-neuropathy-cipn

Nakagaki M, Kennedy GA, Gavin NC, Clavarino A, Whitfield K. The incidence of severe oral mucositis in patients undergoing different conditioning regimens in haematopoietic stem cell transplantation. Support Care Cancer. 2022 Nov;30(11):9141-9149. doi: 10.1007/s00520-022-07328-4. Epub 2022 Aug 26. PMID: 36008731; PMCID: PMC9410738.

Plummer C, Henderson RD, O'Sullivan JD, Read SJ. Ischemic stroke and transient ischemic attack after head and neck radiotherapy: a review. Stroke. 2011 Sep;42(9):2410-8. doi: 10.1161/STROKEAHA.111.615203. Epub 2011 Aug 4. PMID: 21817150.

Pranjic N, Bajraktarevic A, Ramic E. Distress and PTSD in patients with cancer: Cohort study case. Materia socio-medica. 2016;28(1):12. doi: 10.5455/msm.2016.28.12-16.

Raber-Durlacher JE, Barasch A, Peterson DE, Lalla RV, Schubert MM, Fibbe WE. Oral complications and management considerations in patients treated with high-dose chemotherapy. Support Cancer Ther. 2004 Jul 1;1(4):219-29. doi: 10.3816/SCT.2004.n.014. PMID: 18628146.

Salum FG, Medella-Junior FAC, Figueiredo MAZ, Cherubini K. Salivary hypofunction: An update on therapeutic strategies. Gerodontology. 2018 Dec;35(4):305-316. https://doi:10.1111/ger.12353. Epub 2018 Jun 29. PMID: 29956369.

Silver, Julie K. MD; Baima, Jennifer MD. American Journal of Physical Medicine and Rehabilitation, August 2013 – Volume 92, Issue 8, P 715-727, doi:10.1097/PHM.0b013e31829b4afe.

Streckfus, C.F., Bigler, L., Edwards, C., Guajardo-Streckfus, C., Bigler, S.A. (2015). Using Saliva Secretions to Model Disease Progression. In: Streckfus, C. (eds) Advances in Salivary Diagnostics. Springer, Berlin, Heidelberg. doi.org/10.1007/978-3-662-45399-5_9.

Swarm, R. A., Paice, J. A., Anghelescu, D. L., Are, M., Bruce, J. Y., Buga, S., Chwistek, M., Cleeland, C., Craig, D., Gafford, E., Greenlee, H., Hansen, E., Kamal, A. H., Kamdar, M. M., LeGrand, S., Mackey, S., McDowell, M. R., Moryl, N., Nabell, L. M., Nesbit, S., BCPS, O'Connor, N., Rabow, M. W., Rickerson, E., Shatsky, R., Sindt, J., Urba, S. G., Youngwerth, J. M., Hammond, L. J., & Gurski, L. A. (2019). Adult Cancer Pain, Version 3.2019, NCCN Clinical Practice Guidelines in Oncology. Journal of the National Comprehensive Cancer Network J Natl Compr Canc Netw, 17(8), 977-1007. Retrieved Oct 20, 2025, from doi.org/10.6004/jnccn.2019.0038.

Vanhoecke B, De Ryck T, Stringer A, Van de Wiele T, Keefe D. Microbiota and their role in the pathogenesis of oral mucositis. Oral Dis. 2015 Jan;21(1):17-30. doi:10.1111/odi.12224. Epub 2014 Feb 25. PMID: 24456144.

Vega Charles P. MD, Bernard Amy MS, BSN, RN-BC. Understanding the Values and Ethics of Interprofessional Collaboration, CME 2/11/2016; Reviewed and Renewed: 3/8/2017. https://www.medscape.org/viewarticle/857826

Zhang H, Xie M, Archibald SD, Jackson BS, Gupta MK. Association of marijuana use with psychosocial and quality of life outcomes among patients with head and neck cancer. JAMA Otolaryngol Head Neck Surg. 2018 Aug 2. doi: 10.1001/jamaoto.2018.0486

https://dentistry.ucsf.edu/research/cambra

https://www.youtube.com/watch?v=q9kPdQMyU40

https://checkyourmouth.org/wp/

https://oralcancerfoundation.org/

https://www.amazon.com/Get-Your-Spit-Together-checkups/dp/1777716500

https://www.drbicuspid.com/dental-hygiene/oral-systemic-link/cardiovascular/article/15374721/study-reports-epinephrine-safe-in-heart-failure-patients

https://sideeffectsupport.com/

https://www.who.int/cancer/palliative/definition/en/.

https://www.angelsgracehospice.com/hospice-services/hospice-care-comfort-care-whats-the-difference/

https://www.vitas.com/hospice-and-palliative-care-basics/about-palliative-care/hospice-vs-palliative-care-whats-the-difference

https://www.nia.nih.gov/health/what-are-palliative-care-and-hospice-care

ADDITIONAL RESOURCES

UCSF School of Dentistry: https://dentistry.ucsf.edu/research/cambra

Oral Cancer Examination: https://www.youtube.com/watch?v=q9kPdQMyU40

Check Your Mouth: https://checkyourmouth.org/wp/

The Oral Cancer Foundation: https://oralcancerfoundation.org/

Get Your Spit Together!: Your Saliva May Hold the Secret to Better Dental Checkups: https://www.amazon.com/Get-Your-Spit-Together-checkups/dp/1777716500

DrBicuspid: https://www.drbicuspid.com/dental-hygiene/oral-systemic-link/cardiovascular/article/15374721/study-reports-epinephrine-safe-in-heart-failure-patients

Side Effect Support: https://sideeffectsupport.com/

World Health Organization: https://www.who.int/cancer/palliative/definition/en/

Angels Grace: https://www.angelsgracehospice.com/hospice-services/hospice-care-comfort-care-whats-the-difference/

VITAS Healthcare: https://www.vitas.com/hospice-and-palliative-care-basics/about-palliative-care/hospice-vs-palliative-care-whats-the-difference

National Institute on Aging: https://www.nia.nih.gov/health/what-are-palliative-care-and-hospice-care

Dry Mouth and Mucositis Care

Salivary

Substitutes (Rx)

Gelclair

https:/gelclair.com/

SalivaMax (6.25-7.25)

https://forwardscience.com/salivamax

Salube

https://www.ndrugs.com/?s=salube

Salivary Stimulants/Moisturizing/Symptom Relief (Rx or Through Dental Distributor)

3M Xerostomia Relief Spray

https://midwestdental.com/3m-xerostomia-relief-spray-2x10ml-vials

Evoxac (Cervimeline)

https://www.webmd.com/drugs/2/drug-18092/cevimeline-oral/details

Enamelon Preventive Treatment Gel (4.6)

https://www.premierdentalco.com/product/hygien epreventativ e/fluoride/enamelon-preventive-gel/

GC Dry Mouth Gel (7.0)

https://www.gc.dental/america/products/operatory/preventive/gc-dry-mouth-gel

Moisyn

https://periosciences.com/pages/moisyn?srsltid=AfmBOor10E5n2nZgRp104gfXXyNET-sV82mKw3WiPmPZh48f934dUKSM

Mugard

https://mugard.com/

NeutraSal (6.25-7.25)

https://www.webmd.com/drugs/2/drug-153868/neutrasal-mucous-membrane/details#uses

Perio Sciences (7.15)

https://periosciences.com/

SalivaMax

https://forwardscience.com/salivamax

Salagen (pilocarpine)

https://www.webmd.com/drugs/2/drug-78603/pilocarpine-oral/details

Salivary Stimulants/Moisturizing/Symptom Relief (OTC)

Act Lozenges or Rinse (5.7)

https://www.actoralcare.com/en-us/products/lozenges/dry-mouth

All Day Spray/Gel (7.0)

https://www.elevateoralcare.com/products/Allday

Aquoral spray (6.30-6.5)

https://aquoralspray.com/?srsltid=AfmBOopSwBdbFFPIlH2iJOsbZPCjybIYMRFlC8zX9Bw3ICukh37qzh37

Biotene Oral Balance (6-6.7)
https://www.biotene.com/dry-mouth-products/

Bioxtra

https://bioxtra.info/en/products/bioxtra-dry-mouth-oral-gel/.com

ClōSYS 7.1

https://arcadiach.com/oral-care/

Entertainer's Secret (7.0)

https://www.entertainers-secret.com/

Hylamints (4.8)

https://hyalogic.com/search/?q=hylamints

Lumineux Oral Essentials Rinse

https://lumineuxhealth.com/collections/mouthwash

Lubricity (4.0)

https://lubricityinnovations.com/lubricity/

MighTeaFlow (7.37)

https://camellix.com/mighteaflow-2/

Moi-Stir

http://www.moi-stir.com

MouthKote (3.3)

https://www.parnellpharm.com/

Nature's Answer Perio Brite rinse and lozenges (6.5)

https://www.naturesanswer.com/personal-care/oral-care/

Oral B Dry Mouth Rinse

https://oralb.com/en-us/products/compare/rinse/dry-mouth-rinse-moisturizing-mint

Oasis (6.49)

https://www.walmart.com/c/brand/oasis-oral-rinsemouthwash

Spry (7.0)

http://www.xlear.com/

Vega Oral Care (7.0)

https://stellalife.com/products/vega-oral-care-rinse-16oz

Salese Muco-Adhesive disks (8.0)

https://salesedrymouth.com/

Salivea

https://www.salivea.com/why-salivea

Saliva Sure (7.0)

https://www.scandinavianformulas.com/

Smart Mouth Rinse or lozenges (5.5)

https://www.amazon.com/s?k=SmartMouth&me=A2EJCTH67GJMT3&ref=nb_sb_noss

Theramints (7.0)

https://www.solventum.com/en-us/home/v/v000182944/

Tri-ology

https://triologycare.com/products/rinses/

Xerostom (7.0)

https://www.biocosmetics.es/productos

Xylident

https://xylident.co/

Xyligel (7.4)

https://www.oracoat.com/products/xyligel

Xylimelts (8.0)

https://www.oracoat.com/

Remineralization (OTC)

Basic Bites

https://www.basicbites.com/professional/

Remineralization (Rx)

MI Paste One

http://www.gcamerica.com/products/preventive/MI_Paste_ONE/

ReminPro

https://www.voco.dental/us/products/preventive-care/protective-dental-care.aspx

Some products are considered OTC but can only be purchased directly online from the manufacturer—they are not available in a retail store. Others are available to be dispensed

from a dental/medical practitioner's office because they require a prescription.

pH values are given when known. Not all products, depending on their intended use, will have a pH value.

Some products are only available in the United States, Canada, and/or Australia/New Zealand

The information in this appendix is intended for reference purposes. It is not intended, nor should it be interpreted, as medical advice or medical instructions or to replace your doctor's advice. You are advised to consult your own medical doctor(s) for all matters involving your health and medical care. Any reproduction of graphics or content without written permission is not allowed.

About the Author:

Kris Potts, BS, FAADH, RDH is a nationally recognized speaker, oncology-trained dental hygienist, and acted as a Key Opinion Leader for several well-known dental companies. Her passion for patient-centered care was shaped by her own experience as a caregiver and cancer survivor. Through her writing, lectures, and advocacy, Kris empowers dental professionals to become essential partners in the cancer care continuum. When oral health is prioritized, patients face cancer treatment with greater strength, comfort, and dignity.

www.krispottsrdh.com krprdh79@gmail.com

www.ingramcontent.com/pod-product-compliance
Lightning Source LLC
LaVergne TN
LVHW022222200926
848481LV00006B/2086